YES, IT REALLY IS THE FAT!

YES, IT REALLY IS THE FAT!

How I permanently lost 40 pounds in just two months with no pills, no additional exercise, and ABSOLUTELY NO REDUCTION WHATSOEVER in the amount of food that I eat.

Robert J Ruettger

ISBN-13: 9781514818619
ISBN-10: 1514818612
Library of Congress Control Number: 2015911377
CreateSpace Independent Publishing Platform
North Charleston, South Carolina

My Story

The following is the exact, true story of how I personally lost all of my excess weight over six years ago and have almost effortlessly kept it off ever since. This is not meant to be taken as a how-to guide to weight loss. It is simply exactly what happened to me, so take it for what it is worth. If this serves as some sort of useful example, great. I have also tried to keep all of this as short and simple as possible so that it can easily be read multiple times.

The kicker is, I never planned on losing any weight when I started this. It was pretty much an accident. Since about the age of thirty, I have always been about forty pounds overweight. In high school, I was about 175, which is the ideal weight for my height of just under six feet. Around the age of thirty my metabolism slowed down, and my weight gradually climbed to about 215, where it stabilized. Fortunately, even though I consumed a lot of fat, carbs, and sugar, I never gained more than that, but my weight never went down either. I lost weight twice over a twenty-five-year period by exercising like crazy. Both times I kept my weight down to around 175 for about one year before giving up on exercise and gaining every single pound back. My second experience with exercise / weight loss was a killer. I religiously walked over one hour every single day, rain or shine, for almost a year. We're talking a part-time job, which could never last.

Anyway, I pretty much gave up on any hope of losing those forty pounds ever again. For starters, I loved to eat pastry, pizza, cheeseburgers, and potato chips, all of which usually contain tons of fat. I also vehemently hate the idea of anything that remotely suggests a "diet." I have a visceral and psychological hatred of diets. You only live once. Food is meant to be enjoyed. I tried a few diets and could not last on one for more than about twenty-four hours. I felt that diets were unnatural and, worse yet, only temporary solutions. Even if I could tolerate one, I always knew that once I started eating normal food again, I would gain every stinking pound back. So why bother? I always felt that a permanent change in how I ate would be the only way to lose weight and keep it off. By permanent, I mean for the rest of my life. That is not by any description the same thing as a diet.

Anyway, over the years, I attempted to watch the content of fat grams in processed and restaurant food, which is, by the way, most of what I eat. However, I never seriously considered a drastic, permanent, lifelong reduction in my fat intake until about six years ago. By the way, forget about cutting back on sugar, carbs, and sodium. I can't handle it. I'm sorry. I still drink about one liter of full-strength soda every single day. I mean the hard stuff. I do not like water, and I despise all diet sodas. I am trying to change. I know it is immoral and despicable to drink that much high-calorie soda. However, I am also afraid that if I drink less of it, I may lose even more weight. Then there is sodium. If you want to get truly depressed real fast, check out the sodium content in processed foods. We are talking hideous amounts. It is in everything. I mean everything has tons of it. OK, so they use some of it as a preservative. Can't they come up with something else? Then there are the carbs. How I pity anyone who would ever give up bread, pasta, and pastries just to lose weight. That, to me, is deprivation and a true sacrifice. Forget it. I won't do it. I love filling up on my carbs.

2

My High Blood Pressure

About six years ago, at the age of fifty-eight, I went to the doctor and was told that I had high blood pressure and had to start taking medication for it. I was very upset about that, to say the least. I told myself that the very next day, I would make some sort of permanent change to my diet, and then I actually did. Oh, by the way, increasing my exercise like I did before was not much of an option. I work in a home improvement store and as a result walk probably a couple miles every day, when I am not lifting boxes and climbing ladders.

Sorry, I don't have the extra energy for any additional exercise, especially the amount needed to lower blood pressure or lose any substantial amount of weight.

Anyway, I had to decide what part of my diet I could easily alter **with the least amount of sacrifice**. Also, I wanted to keep this very simple and very easy to focus on. Here again, I love food, and we are talking about the rest of my life here, not some stupid temporary diet. This, for me, was an easy decision. Of all the nasty stuff out there, fat means the least to me. To me it is by far the easiest thing for which you can find substitutes that taste just as good. I decided I would miss fat far less than I would ever miss carbs or sugar. If I reduced carbs or sugar, I would be cutting out a lot of food that is filling and satisfying to me and has nowhere near the tasteless calories that fat has.

Make no mistake, tasteless fat is a huge source of calories, not that I ever count calories, because I don't. Also, keep in mind that when it comes to food, I was totally undisciplined. If I can easily make this adjustment, then anyone can.

Fat is everywhere. Americans consume tons of totally unnecessary lard. They are gorging on it. Unfortunately, many food manufacturers and restaurants indiscriminately cram lard into everything whether it adds anything to the taste or not. Also, they have no real incentive to cut back on it. They assume for whatever dumb reason that people will never eat any of their food unless it is loaded with fat. They also, obviously, do not care much about the health of their customers. Some fast-food restaurants that do offer a few low-fat sandwiches actually go out of their way not to advertise those items as being low in fat for fear that customers will avoid them because they surely must not have any taste. The federal guidelines recommend sixty-five grams of dietary fat per day for the average person who consumes about two thousand calories. They're kidding, right? My usual daily consumption of an egg sandwich and fried hash browns in the morning; a cheeseburger, fries, and a fatty pastry for lunch; an occasional candy bar; and pizza for dinner, not to mention the potato chips and ice cream, probably put me around 150 grams of fat on any typical day. Ever try counting your daily intake of fat grams just for fun? Much of this fat is so hidden and adds up so fast. It can all get pretty scary. Not only is it everywhere, but so much of it is so easy to eliminate. Ever check out the fat content in just one bottle of salad dressing made with vegetable oil? You won't believe what's in it, and people think they are eating something that is healthy when they have a salad covered with that dressing. How sad.

Anyway, the day following my blood pressure diagnosis, I started taking one small pill to regulate blood pressure. Since I am used to taking vitamins, one more pill did not seem to be a very big deal. It is worth mentioning, by the way, that I still take this pill even though the whole reason I went low fat was to lower my blood pressure. Even though my typical blood pressure reading is now usually below normal, my doctor has told me to continue taking the medication. I do it only because I don't mind being a little under 120 over 80. Anyway, I do not think he actually believes me when I tell him that I watch my diet. How many times has he heard that one? However, I sure look like I do. By the way, my bad cholesterol reading ten years ago was 145. Now, ten years later at the age of sixty-four, my bad cholesterol is 74! Also, it is worth mentioning that I used to suffer from really nasty episodes of acid reflux about twice a week. This went on every single week for several years. Now I experience it only about once every six months if I happen to eat something that contains a lot of acid, such as tomato sauce, late at night. In other words, my acid reflux was caused almost entirely by a diet that was high in fat. I digress.

The very next day after hearing about my elevated blood pressure, I decided to do only one thing. I wanted to keep this as simple and as painless as possible and limited myself to a daily maximum intake of twenty grams of fat. That is, of course, about one-third of the laughably optimistic sixty-five grams that are recommended daily by the government. This is absolutely the only change that I made in what I eat. I repeat: **This is the only thing that I changed, period**. Also, I decided not to differentiate between "good fat" and "bad fat." I know that some fats are somewhat better for your health than others. Sorry, I have to keep this as simple as possible. To me, fat is fat; I do not care where it comes from. I only make two exceptions to this simple approach. First, I do not eat any trans fats at all, because I believe that they are poison. Also, I try to keep saturated fat at about half my daily fat intake, which is still below what the federal guidelines recommend. That's it, except for one other thing: I almost never weigh myself. I will do it maybe about once every few months. Keep in mind I never went on this permanent low-fat lifestyle to lose weight. That would seem to me to be dangerously close to a "diet," and you know how I feel about diets. I was interested only in improving my health by reducing the amount of lard going into my body and hopefully lowering my blood pressure and maybe my bad cholesterol as well. I did not just "try" this to see whether it worked. Permanently cleansing my system of excess fat was the only objective I had in mind, not losing weight. Weight loss was never ever my primary goal, which is why I never expected to see the excess weight come off as fast as it did. Also, it is very important to keep in mind that many naturally skinny people apparently blessed with very high metabolisms still suffer from high blood pressure and high levels of bad cholesterol.

3

My Weight-Loss Shocker

To be honest, I did think that perhaps maybe as a result of this change in eating habits, I might actually lose a little weight. I would have been very happy if I had shed about ten pounds. Well, near the end of a two-month time period after starting this low-fat lifestyle—and by the way, I stuck to it every single day since I was always thinking only about lowering my blood pressure as opposed to losing weight—I found it to be a lot easier than I ever imagined, and I started having to tighten my belt. A lot. By the way, this weight loss really accelerated toward the end of the second month. Also, keep in mind that two months is not at all a long time to wait if you are not on a "diet" but are rather making a permanent change in what you eat. I never would have even thought of weighing myself any earlier. Finally, after two months I dragged out the old scale and dusted it off. I got on it expecting to see my weight down from 215 to maybe 205 or even 200. Wrong. I weighed exactly 175. I was totally shocked. I almost fell off the scale. Actually, at that point I was sort of scared. The weight had disappeared almost too fast. I immediately increased my daily fat intake to thirty grams, which is where it has stayed ever since. I was afraid of losing any more weight. Anyway, that was almost six years ago. My weight has never ever increased since. In fact, every few months, when my belt seems a little too loose, I weigh myself. My weight has often dropped as low as 165, which is ten pounds under where I should be. How strange it is after being forty pounds overweight for almost thirty years to actually have trouble keeping my weight on. I guess I just have to live with being skinny. Eating more food is not at all an option. I already eat all that I want.

Several people I know, most of them over-weight, like to tell me how evil carbs and sugar are. According to them, carbs and sugar convert to fat. OK, maybe that is true. But what then does fat convert to? Triple fat? These same people also like to get real defensive about the many beneficial attributes of high lard consumption and love telling me that I'm too skinny. Other people will ask me why I continue to limit my fat intake, being as thin as I am. They all have this "temporary diet" mentality. They don't seem to understand that eating a low-fat diet is not just how I got thin. It is also the way I will stay thin for the rest of my life. Keep in mind, I still do eat some fat. I just don't gorge on it like everybody else. Also, it is worth noting that almost the entire nation is obsessed with losing weight, and most of these people never do. Many of these people are totally addicted to fad diets. All they ever want to hear about is "the latest thing." Just cutting out a ton of needless and often tasteless fat seems way too simple. Well, it's that simple. People will also tell me I lost weight only because of my unique metabolism. Yeah, like where was it for the last thirty years when I needed it? Seriously, there is nothing that unique about my metabolism. Anyway, I am still trying to cut back on sugar, especially my soda consumption. It's a wonder they haven't found a way to cram lard into soda. However, I am also afraid that I might have even more trouble keeping my weight on if I do cut back on sugar. Nice problem to have, huh?

4

How I Monitor My Fat Intake

So, how exactly do I keep my daily fat intake at about thirty grams? By the way, there is nothing magical about my choice of thirty grams. A limit of forty or fifty grams of fat may also work fine, but I just happen to be totally comfortable with thirty grams. That's how easy it is for me. I have no desire to eat more fat than that, and it would also be more difficult to keep track of the grams if I ate a higher amount. Anyway, all of this is a lot easier than you may think. Actually, after a while it becomes somewhat of a game. Keep in mind, there are so many countless great-tasting substitutes for tasteless, worthless fat. By the way, why would anybody ever waste their time and sanity counting calories or watching portion sizes, for the rest of their life no less, when the food they are eating is still high in fat? Remember, I used to be a junk food addict. The whole concept of "diet" was totally foreign to me. I love to eat. I love pastries. I eat mostly convenient and microwaveable processed foods. I eat out a lot. I love buffets. None of that has changed at all. I still waddle out of casino and cruise ship buffets so stuffed I can hardly move. Face it, the extra helpings are free. Keep in mind, it is very important to remember that a small portion of food can be loaded with fat and still be far less filling than a much larger portion of food that contains low or even no fat. This larger portion of low-fat food may actually be too much for you to finish! Here again, I never ever count calories or worry about eating smaller portions since I would always be hungry. **I eat all of the food I want. I am never hungry. I have never ever cut back on the actual amount of food that I eat. Never.** That would be a "diet," and **I hate diets**. So, what about dessert? All you need to do is cut the unnecessary fat out of your cakes, icings, brownies, fudge, and pies. If necessary, learn to bake it yourself. For one example, I have learned how to make really great tasting, totally nonfat brownies using fat-free vanilla yogurt instead of oils or milk. Life is short. I eat all the dessert I want. So what do I gorge myself on when I do go to a buffet? I love vegetables, fruit, breaded and nonbreaded food that is baked or grilled as opposed to fried. I eat a lot of fish, chicken, turkey, lean beef, rice, potatoes, pasta, and, of course, shrimp cocktail. However, shrimp is indeed very unusual since it is almost nonfat but still contains a significant amount of cholesterol. Most low-fat food is automatically low in cholesterol. Beware, the reverse is not always true. A lot of low-cholesterol food can still be very high in fat. Anyway, unfortunately a lot of very low-fat seafood is still fairly high in cholesterol. Oh well, life is not always fair. It is worth mentioning, however, that the government is starting to modify its previous concern about any cholesterol in many types of seafood. Also, one final note about buffets is worth mentioning. Beware, the biggest culprits at buffets are the desserts, which are usually needlessly loaded with large amounts of tasteless fat.

One very successful way I have been able to lower my fat intake is when I eat out, which is very often, I do not eat items that I know I can fix at home later without all of the extra fat. This is key. Hot dogs, pudding, yogurt, ice cream, all types of pastry, pasta, pizza, cheeseburgers, nonfried breaded fish and chicken, and all types of low-fat cold-cut sandwiches are among the countless items I can make at home with only about 10 percent of the fat I would normally get in a restaurant. Also included would be fruits, vegetables, soft pretzels, cakes, and dips made with nonfat sour cream, as well as baked french fries. Nothing is more filling, by the way, than a huge salad of lettuce, tomatoes, and low-fat cold cuts topped with nonfat or low-fat cheese and oil-free salad dressing. Some of this stuff when served in restaurants is drowning in unnecessary lard. I avoid it always, and so much of it doesn't even taste that great to begin with, so why eat it? Restaurant appetizers, by the way, are usually the very worst. When eating out, I go for the low-fat entrees, constantly reminding myself that I can always make the other stuff at home. I check the fat content and ask myself whether eating that item is really worth consuming that many grams of fat. Do I really crave it, or is it just more unnecessary, tasteless lard? Even if the high-fat food is on sale at a restaurant or free at a party, I have no trouble skipping it. I can always make a low-fat or nonfat version of it later on at home that tastes every bit as good, if not better. Also, I don't buy the restaurants' excuses for dishing out tons of fat, such as "people come here for special occasions, and a little extra fat won't hurt." No way, it's not just "a little extra fat," and people eat out at those places constantly.

Not long ago I checked the fat content in one apple pie made at the bakery of a local grocery store. I mean, just how difficult is it to ruin something as supposedly healthy as apple pie? Well, the fat content of that one pie was about two hundred grams, not to mention their cakes. I'm not sure, but I think their cake icing may be made with motor oil. You almost have to use paint thinner to get what's left off the dish. I obviously avoid most grocery store–prepared foods. No one needs to consume all of this useless, tasteless lard. I do not miss it at all. I have actually over time developed a real aversion to unnecessary fat and lard. I also tend to resent it when restaurants, or anyone else for that matter, try to cram tasteless fat on me. Here again, it usually doesn't taste any better than a much lower fat option, so why should I eat it?

5

Great-Tasting Low-Fat Substitutes

When I decided to increase my daily fat intake from twenty grams to thirty grams to avoid losing any more weight, I really wasn't sure I actually wanted to. I didn't miss the fat. The bottom line is there are so many great-tasting substitutes for fat. If I felt it was any real sacrifice, I could never do it for more than a couple days, let alone for the past six years. Fortunately, for me anyway, food labels exist. I know that the fat content listed is not always exactly accurate, but I would be totally lost without knowing how much fat is in all of the food I buy in grocery stores or consume at my favorite restaurants, especially when some of the fat content listed occasionally comes as a real shock. A lot of this is common sense. In the absence of actual labels, I have also become an expert at "rating" a meal, which means giving myself a good estimate of the fat content based on past experience. After a while one gets pretty good at this. In addition, when I am at home, I mark down the approximate grams of fat that I have eaten that day on an index card, which sure is a lot simpler than trying to count calories. Also, what about the occasional days when I consume significantly more than thirty grams of fat? This may happen to me on average about once a month, at holiday celebrations, weddings, whatever. It happens to even the best of us. If I have a day when I know I've gone well over thirty grams, I just reduce my fat intake to about ten or fifteen grams the next day or two to make up for it. For me this is ridiculously easy to do. However, these lapses almost never occur, because I don't crave any of this high-fat food when I know I can substitute something else that I like every bit as much. Also, keep in mind, organic foods, natural foods, and so-called nonprocessed foods can be a real problem. Here again, common sense prevails. **"Organic" and "natural" do not necessarily mean "low fat."** Many health-food and natural-food items are still loaded with tasteless fat. On the other hand, some fast-food and processed-food entrees can actually be very low in fat. I am not a natural-food snob. I prefer being skinny. Also, many salad dressings and other foods that are labeled "low fat" or, worse yet, "lite" are actually loaded with fat! Read the labels, and also do not take the restaurant server's word for it. I also avoid packaged snack foods that say "lite." They are usually just serving miniature versions or "bite-size" portions of the very same high-fat snack you would normally get in their regular size packages. Why bother? **I do not want less food or smaller portions.** I want normal portions with less fat! I'm hungry!

I constantly look at fat content. I don't care who makes it or where it comes from; if it's full of useless lard, I don't want it. Labels that claim "natural," "healthy," or "organic" mean absolutely nothing to me if it's also high in fat. Also, beware, it is often very easy to think that one fast-food item sounds healthier than another until you look at the fat content and realize that the reverse is actually true. One restaurant might make healthy and great-tasting low-fat chili, pasta sauces, or pancakes, and another restaurant that doesn't care will pump in the extra tasteless, worthless lard. By the way, all of this restaurant nutritional information is easily accessible on the Internet. Just be prepared for some surprises, both good and bad. Also, beware that for some idiotic reason a lot of the new food labels are starting to focus only on saturated fat grams. Although saturated fat is an important thing to watch, I count **total fat grams**, not just saturated. **Remember, it is actually quite easy to eat very little saturated fat and cholesterol while still consuming a very high amount of total fat.** If I had continued to gorge myself on all of the so-called good fats while limiting only my intake of saturated fat, I know for a fact that I would never have lost over forty pounds, my bad cholesterol probably would not have been cut in half, and I obviously would not be writing this book. Sorry, I still believe that fat is fat no matter where it comes from.

6

Keep It Simple

In closing, as I said earlier, this is not meant to be just another how-to guide to weight loss. Yes, I want to share this information with others so that they may see some value in this approach. However, I just wanted to report what actually happened to me in real life and why I truly believe that excess fat intake is, by far, the biggest culprit when it comes to obesity, far more important than carbs or even sugar. Recently this constant war on carbs and sugar seems to be all that I have been hearing about. Cutting carbs and sugar would be to me a starvation diet, a huge sacrifice, and something that could never be maintained for a person's entire lifetime. Why is so little attention being paid to fat, and more specifically vegetable oil? It doesn't matter where it comes from, whether it is "good oil" or "bad oil"; all vegetable oil is loaded with fat. The same can also be said for basically all nuts. At least high-fat butter and mayonnaise have some flavor. On the other hand, almost-tasteless vegetable oil is used everywhere and is often also used as a substitute for dairy products, possibly because of its longer shelf life. Check out the huge fat content in one small can of cake icing. Make your own homemade cake icing! Use sugar, skim milk, nonfat yogurt, nonfat sour cream, anything other than oil. Just remember, any processed food or snack that contains any kind of oil, vegetable or otherwise, automatically contains totally unnecessary and almost-tasteless fat. Skip it. You will almost never miss it if you leave it out. If you want to cut back on fat, you have to avoid, or at the very least greatly reduce, your reliance on all oils. Everyone knows it is the oil that makes fried food so fattening. It doesn't matter if it's "good oil" or "bad oil." Well, guess what. It has the same exact effect on everything else.

Remember the apple pie that I mentioned earlier that had about two hundred grams of fat? Obviously, for an apple pie one needs to include apples, cinnamon, flour, and sugar, all of which are fat-free. All you need to do is cut out or at least greatly reduce the butter and oils and use other ingredients instead, such as nonfat yogurt, nonfat milk, nonfat sour cream, or nonfat egg whites. At the very least, use some type of fat/

nonfat combination. Is the perfect superflakey pie crust worth all of that extra fat? Personally, I can easily skip the extra flakes and the two hundred grams of fat that go with it. This same approach also goes for any other recipe you can think of. If you can't totally eliminate the fat, combine it with something else that is nonfat. Need extra cheese on your pizza? I use nothing but nonfat shredded cheese, but you could also combine an equal amount of nonfat cheese with your other regular cheese. This way you will at least cut your total fat in half. However, it is worth mentioning, I am by no means recommending a high-carb or high-sugar diet for anyone. I believe if one thinks for whatever reason that it is important to also cut down on carbs, sugar, portion amounts, calories, sodium, or gluten, just to name a few (gee, I'm already worn out just thinking about it), and if you really want to constantly monitor all of that for the rest of your life, fine. It's no wonder most people put all of this off. **However, I also believe that without a big reduction in the amount of worthless, tasteless, and totally unnecessary lard that one takes in, it is all a complete waste of time.** Fat is a hugely powerful source of calories. Why waste so many calories on it? Don't be fooled by the old excuse that you need all of that fat for extra energy. No normal person needs to take in that much fat. I firmly believe if you do not cut back substantially on fat consumption, you will never ever achieve any permanent weight loss or any other lasting health benefits. Keep in mind that cutting back on excess fat is such a simple concept and so easy to focus on. Also, forget about all of the so-called experts and not-so-slim celebrities who tell you to load up on "good fat." Remember how these same experts used to push trans-fat margarine? Fat is fat. Do I sound just a little militant here? Never mind the fact that these experts as well as many public officials and members of the media, keep relentlessly pounding on the idea that sugar is public enemy number one, some of them actually wanting to ban it, while they blissfully ignore the fact that the entire country is drowning in fat. Ever wonder how many of these people have actually had the enormous amount of self-discipline it would take to experience substantial and permanent weight loss by only cutting back on sugar? Given this massive media blitz against sugar as well as those equally evil carbs, you would think that by now millions of Americans would finally be losing a lot of excess weight. Well, guess what. They're not. Here again, I'm not pushing the idea of high sugar consumption, but I am recommending what I feel is a far more realistic approach that can be maintained for the rest of one's life. Face it, for most people that would be a rather long time to go without sugar.

Most everyone has heard about the classic stereotype of the poor overweight person ordering their diet soda at a restaurant along with a greasy double cheeseburger and an order of fries. Well, I will personally continue to enjoy my full-strength sugary soda (with refill) along with my grilled-chicken sandwich topped with nonfat barbecue sauce or honey mustard, or my low-fat ham-and-turkey sandwich topped with nonfat salad dressing or nonfat mayonnaise, as well as my baked beans or baked potato covered with low-fat chili, not to mention my sugar-coated rice cakes, nonfat cookies, nonfat yogurt, or my nonfat ice cream covered with nonfat syrup. I really am trying hard to cut back on the soda, honest. By the way, honey mustard is a very interesting case in point. Honey mustard, which is to me a great substitute for regular mayonnaise, is almost always totally fat-free. However, for some dumb reason some restaurants actually serve honey mustard that is made with vegetable oil. You know what that does. There is absolutely no reason whatsoever to use it. This is just another example of how ridiculously easy it is to cut out totally unnecessary fat but only if you know what to look for.

One thing I will never ever do is subject myself to any type of temporary "diet," which means eating less food instead of a totally permanent reduction in unhealthy fat and, as a result, bad cholesterol. Many people go on restrictive diet plans thinking that somehow if the weight finally does come off, they will in some way make some kind of magical adjustment in eating habits that will enable them to start eating normally again without gaining every single pound back. They'll worry about how to do that later if they can only get through this awful diet and the weight actually comes off. Losing the weight is their only focus, not keeping it off **forever**. They will cross that bridge when they come to it. Sorry, it doesn't work that way. **You must ask yourself up front, before any weight-loss attempt even starts: Exactly how is that going to happen?** If you can't answer that, don't fool yourself and skip all of the torture. "Diets" are not permanent solutions, period. **Whatever you do has to be a permanent lifelong adjustment from the very first day, something that you feel totally comfortable doing for the rest of your life.** If it isn't, then don't bother, don't waste your time, don't set yourself up for a huge letdown later on.

By only counting fat grams, I eat all the food that I want. My biggest problem now is keeping my weight on. If I eat less food on any given day because I do not feel well or just have no time to eat, I can feel my weight dropping. I had a choice to make. Either I could count calories and watch portion sizes and therefore eat less food and always be hungry for the rest of my life, while still consuming highly caloric and unhealthy fat, or I could cut the fat significantly and still eat all of the food I wanted. Some choice. Also, can you imagine how futile it would be to go on some sort of deprivation low-calorie diet and still end up with high levels of blood pressure and bad cholesterol? Here again, I have to stress repeatedly that I did all of this only for health reasons. My primary goal, ironically, was never weight loss. It just happened. The best advice that I can possibly give you is to count your daily intake of fat grams for just a few days and then decide where you can start almost effortlessly making cuts in the amount of worthless fat you now consume. Hopefully, if you decide to follow my example, you will actually have fun doing it. Coming up with great-tasting substitutes for useless fat has been for me somewhat of a game, which is why I have been able to continue doing it for over six years. Also, thinking how this influences my long-term health has always been my main concern. Need I mention what a really great feeling it is to eat a large pizza topped with lean pepperoni, mushrooms, and a lot of extra cheese (most of it nonfat) and not have to feel guilty about it? Better yet, how about the kick I get looking down at my huge grilled dinner at one of my favorite restaurants, with all of the side dishes I've selected, and realizing that the entire meal has almost no grams of fat in it whatsoever? Then there is the person who is sitting at the table next to me whose small side salad, which is drowning in oil-based dressing, probably has more fat on it than I have eaten in the last two days. I think you get the picture. Just always try to remember: if you don't want to be fat, then **don't eat it!**

Disclaimer

This publication contains the opinions and ideas of its author. It is intended to provide helpful and informative material on the subjects addressed in the publication. It is sold with the understanding that the author and publisher are not engaged in rendering medical, health, or any other kind of personal professional services in the book. The reader should always consult his or her medical, health, nutritional, or other competent professional before adopting any of the suggestions in this book or drawing any inferences from it. This book is not intended to diagnose, treat, cure, or prevent any health problem or condition, nor is it intended to replace the advice of a physician. No action should be taken solely on the book's contents. The author and publisher specifically disclaim all responsibility for any liability, loss, or risk, personal or otherwise, which is incurred as a consequence, directly or indirectly, of the use and application of any of the contents of this book.

Author Robert J. Ruettger